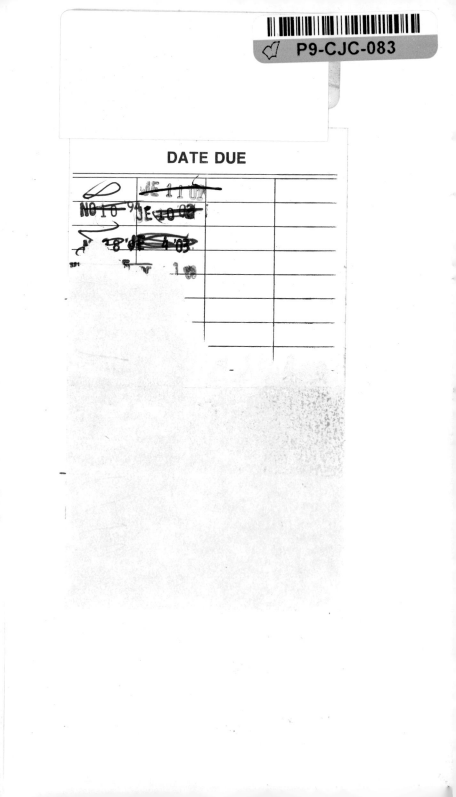

Dyslexia

How Would I Cope?

of related interest

Checkmate
A Pocket-Size Guide to Everyday Spellings for Dyslexics
Alan O'Brien
1 85302 165 2

Children with Special Needs
Assessment, Law and Practice – Caught in the Act
H Chasty and J Friel
1 85302 096 6

Dyslexia
How Would I Cope?

Michael Ryden

with an introduction by Derek Copley

Jessica Kingsley Publishers
London and Philadelphia

First edition published in 1989
Second, revised edition published in 1992 by
Jessica Kingsley Publishers
118 Pentonville Road
London N1 9JB

copyright © 1989 and 1992 Michael Ryden

Cover by Melissa J. Reagan.

British Library Cataloguing in Publication Data

Ryden, Michael
   Dyslexia: How Would I Cope?. - 2Rev.ed
   I. Title
   616.85

ISBN 1-85302-154-7

Printed and bound in Great Britain by
Bookcraft L td., Avon.

Contents

PART III – Attitude Counselling and Teaching

Appendices

Foreword

I count it a privilege to write the foreword to this book.

I have known the author personally for several years and during that time I have observed his determination to succeed in life despite his disability.

I have worked with several dyslexics over the span of my teaching career but Mike was the first one to enable me to step into his shoes and to see things from inside his personal world. He did this not merely by telling me but by showing me, using the experiments described in Part II. It was a real eye opener, and gave me a new sympathetic understanding.

The world has many disabled people, many of whom have come to terms with their limitations and whose self esteem is high. Alas the same is not so true of us who meet disadvantaged people from time to time. We simply do not know how to react and our fears cause us to reject them or treat them with less than the dignity they deserve. We do them a disservice, damage their self image and indeed hinder their progress.

Today there are numerous books written by sufferers of various kinds and, compared with a previous generation, we are much more aware of their difficulties. Television, too, with its honest interviews and documentaries has done much to enlighten us concerning those members of society who suffer.

I have seen very few books which are written for ordinary members of the public on the subject of dyslexia. I therefore commend this book to you in the hope that it will enable you to form genuine friendships with the many Mike Rydens of this world.

Derek Copley

Acknowledgements

Thank you to all who have considered my work for what it is and did not condemn or rebuff me for my lack of reading ability and even more to those who have accepted my short-comings and have helped me by reading to me and giving me the confidence to keep trying to learn how to cope better.

Special thanks to my family for their support and patience in my studies.

Finally thanks to all who do not judge someone, whatever the problem, before they know the abilities of the person concerned.

Michael Ryden
London 1989

Give Me a Chance

by Mike Ryden – a dyslexic

Do I smell because I cannot read?

Socially they rebuff me, maybe because they don't know
how to handle it themselves and it seems especially hard
to share the good things in life. If you can't read,
you are by implication stupid
and therefore not worth bothering with.

I ask you, is reading so all important? Believe me, it is
certainly hard not being able to read
– but is it the only way to communicate?

Would you ask a blind person to look at a photograph,
or take a deaf person to an orchestral concert?

So why disregard me as useless because I cannot read?

Can you do everything?

Give me a fair chance – a fair one is all I ask for,
no more, no less.

Accept me for the person I am,
and for the things that I can do.

Are any of us perfect?

PART I

What is Dyslexia?

Introduction

In today's society one's whole life style is based on reading – from finding street directions and shopping, to checking what is on the TV or radio, and trying to keep up with local and world news.

In the workplace, there is now an excessive amount of paperwork and many forms to be dealt with – even where manual jobs which really require no litercy skills are concerned. One's ability to fill in forms seems to be measured, rather than one's ability to do the job or even one's intelligence.

This book is by no means intended to be an in-depth study of the causes of and possible treatments for learning difficulties, but is intended to create an awareness of the experience of dyslexia – taken from the experience of some other dyslexics as well as my own.

My aim is to cultivate the attitude of parents, teachers and employers, to provide them with the knowledge necessary to understand how a dyslexic is affected, and show them how to concentrate on the dyslexic's strong points so as to minimise the effects of dyslexia.

There are various ways and means of both testing and teaching the dyslexic which require a minimum of effort from teachers, employers and governing bodies.

For example, it is not necessary to write an essay to test a manual skill, and in a workshop the student may do a satisfactory job even though he or she is unable to give an explanation of the process in writing.

*   *   *

What is Dyslexia?

Although the centre of the thought system of the dyslexic is functioning well in most cases, the ability of one or both of the input (obtaining information) or output (imparting information) modes is impaired in some way.

COMMUNICATING – the problem is to find a form or method of communication that is accessible to all parties concerned, and that results in the least impairment or distortion of information. This method, by implication will be the one that is most efficient.

TESTING – where it is possible to give a person tests or examinations in the mode (information format) that best re-creates the working environment, such a test provides a far more realistic assessment of their skills than a purely written test.

In a woodwork class, for example, give the student a joint to make, and ask him or her to just include short notes where absolutely necessary, rather than asking for the task to be described in essay form.

It is estimated that over 10% of the population suffers from dyslexia to some extent, and that about four people in every hundred need special help.

Dyslexia is a genuine difficulty that occurs irrespective of intelligence, but the problems it causes can largely be overcome by the right teaching, understanding, encouragement and support for the determination of the person with dyslexia.

It is not possible for a layman to give advice on the diagnosis and treatment of dyslexia – each individual will have different problems and will need to cope with them in different ways. However, the following section is intended to give some general indication of how dyslexia may show itself.

Recognising dyslexia

Dyslexia can show itself in many ways, including the following:

In writing and reading

- poor concentration or inaccuracy in reading and spelling

- a tendency to put letters or figures the wrong way round, and to reverse their order (for example, b for d, 6 for 9, 48 for 84, raw for war)

- reading a word correctly and then failing to recognise it further down the page

- ability to answer questions orally, but difficulty in writing down the answer

- spelling the same word in several different ways without recognising the correct spelling

- difficulty in copying written work

- difficulty in taking notes

- difficulty in understanding time and tense

- difficulty in working with serial numbering.

In other ways

- being bright in many ways but with an apparent block in others

- confusing left and right

- ambidexterity

- difficulty in carrying out a sequence of instructions

- unusual clumsiness or poor co-ordination

- being far better at answering questions orally than in writing

- hyperactivity, particularly in learning situations

- difficulty in getting sequences in the right order, such as months of the year, or the alphabet.

Characteristics

Many dyslexic children display more than one of the
following characteristics:

- hyperactive

- needs less sleep than the average child

- easily distracted (possibly seeing too much all at
  once rather than not paying attention)

- untidy and disorganised

- poor motor coordination.

*   *   *

It would appear to be a great relief when the problem is
diagnosed and the child not only knows that he or she is
not the only one with this problem, but that what is
causing the trouble actually has a name.

Try to imagine yourself accomplishing everyday tasks
without the skills which you take for granted.

It is important to remember that these characteristics are not necessarily indicative of dyslexia, and that a professional diagnosis should be sought.

*   *   *

It is important to have professional advice as soon as possible, and this should be available through the local education authorities. Under the 1981 Education Act children with special needs should, in theory, get appropriate help – in practice, only two or three Local Education Authorities (LEAs) provide properly trained teachers for dyslexics. LEAs can assess, but it is unlikely that schools will offer appropriate teaching – and remedial teaching is not sufficient. The teacher must be trained in dyslexia and multi-sensory techniques. The majority of parents still have to resort to private teachers. The earlier that help is given, the better the chance of success in minimising the effects of dyslexia.

Within guidelines, the children should be allowed to make their own decisions as far and as early as possible, because it will become more difficult for them to rely on outside help as they get older. With age, also, comes embarrassment at still not being able to read.

PART II

How Does it Feel?

This section provides examples of just how distorted written information can become to a dyslexic.

Text used is about a river trip – written by the author of this book and subsequently published.

Concept reversal

It will been nearly one hundred and twenty days before Minor John Wesley Powell broak history sell follerwing an experdition around the cataract of the Small Canyon. Faced apart seemingly easy evens – some physical, none supernatural – Powell challenged the Colorado flow…

It has been almost one hundred and twenty years since Major John Powell made history by leading an expedition through the cataract of the Grand Canyon. Faced with seemingly insurmountable odds – some physical, some natural – Powell challenged the Colorado river…

Sometimes a dyslexic will perceive the meaning of a word or phrase as its exact opposite.

Vertical disorientation

anddshe was eqAlly adeht at rafting in rhe gad le boat.
ulong sitp ynn, onother pataplegic preeg lwho hrsfthe
uwe ofLonly ane arm)and sevgra(othea reinds n they
pfddle adroitlt theough eiery sapid a,d went aor the big
wayer whrrever vt war.

and she was equally adept at rafting in the paddle boat.
Along with Lynn, another paraplegic Gregg (who has the
use of only one arm) and several other friends, they
paddled adroitly through every rapid and went for the
big water wherever it was.

Letters, or whole words, may appear to be in the line above or below.

Lateral disorientation

humand spirof intere.test Wef ita nda namileWh culties
mustdiff havef acquestuion eth haveseds noe toram ithw
,allenchedynolgni ot mrnaun ethe all dame tedlyuod saw
eatrg casueeb rmoe eth tunforateun ciCivel raW sihaof
diccanet.

a test of human spirit and integrity. While few question
the difficulties he must have faced having only one arm to
work with, the challenge undoubtedly was made all the
more great because of his unfortunate Civil War accident.

*Here words or parts of word appear in the wrong place –
sometimes the letters appearing in reverse order – along a
line*

Fading

after the boats were pulled ashore for lunch or for the
night, the wheelchairs were unloaded first so the students
could take care of setting up tents and getting into dry
clothes.

after the boats were pulled ashore for lunch or for the
night, the wheelchairs were unloaded first so the students
could take care of setting up tents and getting into dry
clothes.

*The first few letters may seem clear and then others fade
until they are barely discernible. This is random fading,
appearing as anything between 20 and 100 dot (full black)*

Mirror image

On the San Juan river in southern Utah just a few
months ago, a special group of NAU students faced a
challenge equally as great. Six eager and energetic
disabled students, five relying on wheelchairs for their
primary means of locomotion, participated in a weekend
river trip of

On the San Juan river in southern Utah just a few
months ago, a special group of NAU students faced a
challenge equally as great. Six eager and energetic
disabled students, five relying on wheelchairs for their
primary means of locomotion, participated in a weekend
river trip of

Text may appear completely reversed, as though it were
being seen in a mirror

Omitting letters

apoxmately thity mles bteen Bluff and Mexcan Ht, Utah.
Althogh the San Jan has been mpped and the eqipmnt hs
impved sine Pwells adeture, for thse studnts, the adenture
ws no lss grat.

approximately thirty miles between Bluff and Mexican
Hat, Utah. Although the San Juan has been mapped and
the equipment has improved since Powell's adventure,
for these students, the adventure was no less great.

Random letters may be omitted.

Omitting words (telegraph style)

It not been that diabled people oppertunity explore remote wild. Prejudice attertuides responsibility barries people willing risk adventure progressive administrators

It has not been long that disabled people have had the opportunity to explore and enjoy remote wild areas. Prejudice and attitudes about responsibility have served as barriers to these people who are willing to take risks and enjoy adventure. But progressive administrators like Linda Price

> *Whole words may be omitted, leaving only the key words.*

Omitting key words

Student services at the, and AL director of Educational Program, are all that. With the of people like of Flagstaff Parks and Department and of the river trip are changing and are relizing.

Disabled Student Services at the university, and Al Jamieson, director of NAU's Educational Support Program, are changing all that. With the help of people like Mark Grant of the Flagstaff Parks and Recreation Department and leader of the trip, attitudes are changing and people are realising

---

Key words may be omitted.

Inversions

that the four-walled classroom is not the limit to
education. The spirit and integrity of the students who
participate in this trip is unrivalled to any yet witnessed.
Helen, head cook for the trip, prepared an elegant menu
– steak, oysters, shrimp omelets

that the four-walled classroom is not the limit to
education. The spirit and integrity of the students who
participate in this trip is unrivalled to any yet witnessed.
Helen, head cook for the trip, prepared an elegant menu
– steak, oysters, shrimp omelets

Text may actually appear to be upside down.

Horizontal reversal

In order to have some idea of the problem PLEASE take two or three minutes to try the following experiment.

Hold a mirror at eye level reflecting double lined shapes. Looking ONLY through the mirror draw a line between the existing ones, using all three shapes.

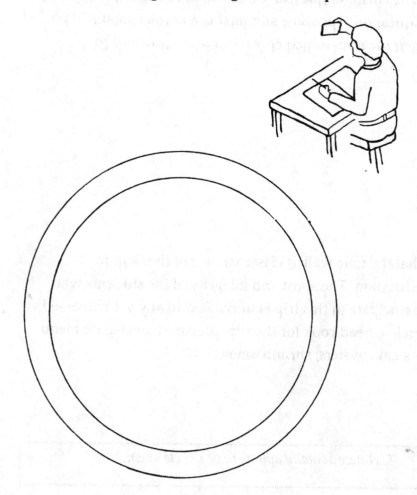

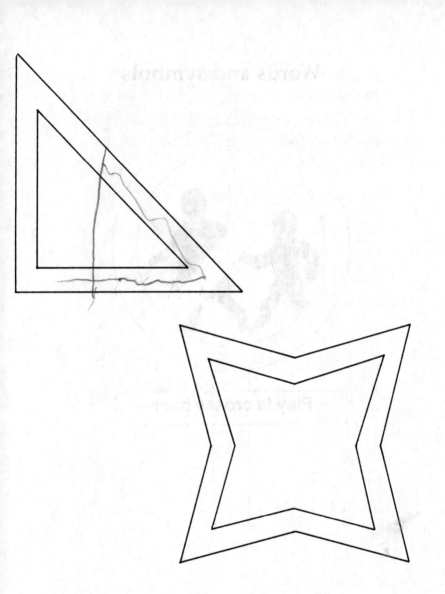

Having finished this experiment you may now have some indication of the feelings of frustration felt by many dyslexics who actually do see things in this way some of the time.

Words and symbols

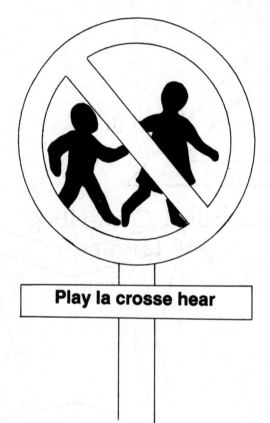

Play la crosse hear

The words describing familiar symbols may appear meaningless, or have quite a different meaning

PART III

Learning, Counselling and Teaching

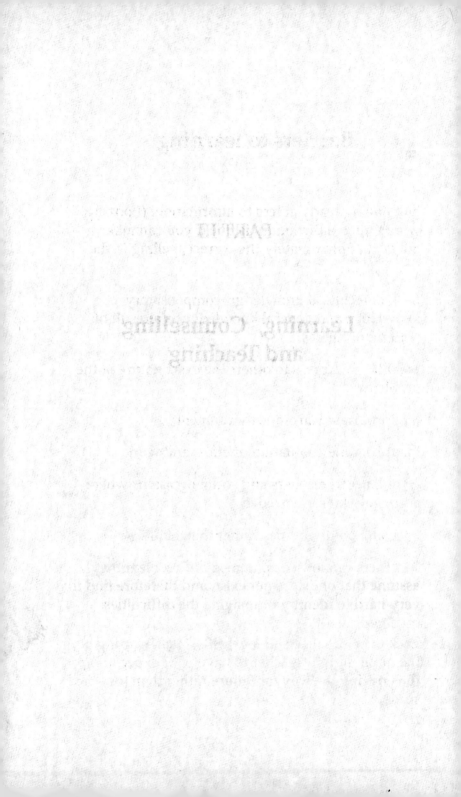

Barriers to learning

- Not having ready access to information. (Looking words up in a dictionary is fine if you can make a guess at approximately the correct spelling in the first place.)

- Lack of technical knowledge, compensatory knowledge and general knowledge as a result of reading problems.

- Inability to express to others the exact nature of the problem.

- Inappropriate learning environment.

- Inappropriate evaluation of effort and work.

- Avoidance of teachers and social occasions where academic skills are needed.

- Focusing on disabilities rather than abilities.

- As others cannot see an immediate problem they assume that one does not exist, and therefore find it very hard to identify or imagine the difficulties involved.
- Lack of confidence and low self-esteem, causing both the pupil and the teacher to have poor expectations – thus paving the way for failure rather than for success.

Commonly recurring attitudes

From teachers and peers:

- Inferior

- Thick (*give up, you'll never make it*)

- Slow (*take your time, you will understand it eventually*)

- Mentally ill (*because you cannot understand in this particular format*)

- Incorrect (*retribution*)

Learning disabled *versus* peers

- Better orally

- Good conceptual memory

- Misuse of words

- Distractive techniques used by the learning disabled

- Slow to answer – even though knowing the answer

- 'Forgetting' homework

- Taking 'the easy way out'

- Pretending to be dumb

- Class clown

Feelings

- Absolutely frustrated with the inability to get through to others coherently – sense of inadequacy

- Wanting to give up

- Angry – furious to the point where sequential thought breaks up at random

- Want to get physically aggressive towards teachers and others

- Having to fight back all the time

- Unfair – persecuted – always being on the defensive

- Isolation – totally and utterly alone

- Rushed – panic

- Escape to an area of ability

- Maybe I am stupid after all (despite a fairly high I.Q.)?

- Is it worth it all?

Finally, to move forward, there must be

- Acceptance of one's disability

- Recognition and use of one's abilities.

*   *   *

There is little stability in a dyslexic's world, for not only the severity but also the form of their problem alters on a daily basis, and there are a tremendous number of symbols which we are all exposed to daily which dyslexics cannot fully understand – this further adds to their confusion and frustration and increases their problems.

It has been shown that many dyslexic students can understand words just as well if they hold the text at right angles or even upside down, as though the shape is more important than the symbol.

Statements made by dyslexics

'My hands don't do what my brain tells them to.'

'My brain will not always do what I want it to.'

'It is impossible to write down what I am thinking – it comes out wrong.'

'Some days I can read reasonably well – other days not at all.'

'I can only manage to read for short periods.'

'I feel completely exhausted when I have read some- thing.'

*   *   *

There seems to be a connection which is especially strong in dyslexics, whereby stress, health and the emotions have a direct bearing on reading ability. Even when a dyslexic has achieved great progress, stress, tiredness, or a particular emotional state can have a temporary effect on the quality of written work.

A common social cycle

The dyslexic meets a stranger who has no knowledge of dyslexic problems; the dyslexic feels inadequate and apprehensive and thus withdraws, and this is followed by rejection on both sides.

This cycle forces many dyslexics to become 'LONERS' and therefore to feel very isolated.

Counselling dyslexia

Comments on 'Barriers', 'Attitudes', 'Feelings' (The counsellor had no prior knowledge that the emotions, barriers and feelings were dyslexic related.)

As a counsellor the areas that I would cover in depth would be:

- Conduct
- Disorder
- Acting out
- Behaviour
-

Suggestions

(a) Find out what the source of their anger, frustration, and hostility is.

(b) Teach appropriate coping strategies to replace the inappropriate ones (i.e. acting-out behaviour).

Q. How would you handle the client?

A. Ask what the specific problems are. Listen with empathy, and try to understand the underlying emotions. Become more aware of their disabilities through research. Help them to understand and cope with their problems and inherent disabilities.

Q. How would you want others to respond to them?

A. They should be aware of the problem but treat the dyslexic as they would a normal person.

They should focus on the dyslexic's abilities and capitalise on those.

Q. What would you do with the released emotions related to the problem?

A. Encourage the person to develop their abilities, thus increasing their self-confidence (focusing on other things). Teach the person how to accept their frustrations, as they will always be with them.

Advice for teaching and learning

- See that the teacher is made aware of the person who has the problem, preferably by a person of authority as well as by the student him or herself.

- Find the best mode of learning for that student.

- Explore different formats for testing (i.e. verbal input/output, diagrammatically, or even manually).

Teaching

It is most useful for a student to be able to select – from information available at the advice centre – the teacher whose method of teaching is most compatible with the student's mode of learning.

This can be done by taking the student/teacher assessment report, and including a question on the predominant mode by which the teachers conveys the subject information to the students.

This should relieve some of the stresses on both teachers and students caused by the lack of communication, and thus create a far more efficient educational system for the dyslexic.

Practical Help

- Allow tape recorders in classes – particularly lectures – and accept students' taped work.

- Allow the use of computers and word processors.

Writing

Computers and word processors are most useful instruments for the dyslexic, for once they have got the bulk of the text programmed into the machine, it can be edited and organised by a non-dyslexic and then retrieved again as and when required by the dyslexic. This is far more helpful than the old method of repetitive rewriting which continuously created more and more mistakes.

However, the spell checker (with or without the computer) is similar to a dictionary, where one must know either the approximate or the phonetic spelling. A dyslexic frequently cannot differentiate between slightly different spellings of words which may have completely different meanings – and which would not be shown up by using a spell checker.

Note taking

The use of underlining and abbreviations is all very well, but until the dyslexic has found his or her own forms and methods of note taking – helped and guided by others – it is necessary that he or she be allowed to pick out what is important and what 'memory joggers' are useful to them rather than to teachers or others concerned.

For example, the study notes must be precise and in a logical sequence for the learning disabled to grasp, and need to be checked for accuracy of content, rather than for the layout and format of the notes – dyslexics cannot check for themselves as preconceptions can and frequently do come into play.

Time and effort

Whilst teaching the correct use and management of time is very important to enable the student to achieve effective output of work, an element of constant encouragement should be given. Unless there is some form of recognition of EFFORT as well as achievement, the student will unquestionably be tempted to neglect those subjects in which they persistently receive zero response.

Communication of ideas

Mere repetition is not necessarily useful in the explanation of a concept or idea in the form in which it was first presented – it may be better to approach from a different angle which the dyslexic may more readily understand. For example, an auditory learner may not be able to read and understand written concepts at all, so written repetition would be useless, and a few extra minutes taken at this time may help to solve the problem of communication – and thus save valuable time in correcting mistakes and misunderstandings.

After all, one would not attempt to teach a blind student solely from the blackboard, so why a dyslexic? Whilst the teacher is writing the question, it should also be read out loud.

In business it may be more beneficial to all, in the long term, to explain an instruction directly, rather than leave a dyslexic to read and work it out for themselves, as many serious mistakes can be caused by the misunderstanding or reversal of a single word or phrase. Once the concept is grasped, often the dyslexic is very good at the intuitive use and interpretation of the instructions.

For the dyslexic there cannot be too much emphasis on

- tell

- demonstrate

- list key concepts

- question to assess correct intake

- and also on allowing the learner to tell, demonstrate, repeat key concepts and practice.

Learning

There must exist a strong desire to learn, especially in the older student – and it is important that the content of the books and articles used be of interest to the age group concerned. There is nothing more humiliating for a ten-year-old than to be given a reader for five-year-olds about the cat sitting on the mat.

If books can be related to the student's interest in sport or a hobby, for example, it will help to keep them involved with reading outside school hours, and provide great motivation.

Probably the most useful fact which dyslexics should be made aware of is that life is not fair, and that they will just have to work that much harder and persevere that much more than the average person, to obtain results comparable with those of people without handicaps.

This awareness will be necessary as the dyslexic gets older, and will be essential – together with the extra drive needed, to compete successfully in the workplace.

*   *   *

Appendices

Appendices

History of Dyslexia

It appears that dyslexia was first diagnosed in 1895 by Dr James Hinshelwood from Glasgow. He stated that a 'very intelligent boy of twelve was unable to learn to read, but had all the lessons in the class been oral lessons, he would probably have been the brightest boy.'

In 1924 – Dr Samuel Orton, an American neuropsychiatrist, began research backed by the Rockefeller Foundation.

In November 1979 – an article in the Boston Globe publicised neurological research work at the Beth Israel Hospital which claimed discovery of physical evidence which showed distinct abnormalities in brain cell structure. This was the work of Dr Anthony Galaburda and Dr Thomas Kemper, neurologists at Beth Israel.

In 1988 – for the first time ever, a student was allowed to use a word processor to take a GCSE examination (*Daily Express, 13th June 1988*)

Experts seem to give various reasons (somewhat unconvincingly) as to why there has been such scant correlation between the educational and neurological fields, and it is to be hoped that, in the light of new discoveries, this particular situation will improve rapidly.

People

Some of the well known people who have succeeded in their chosen careers in spite of their learning disability problems:

Thomas Edison: Thought mentally slow by his teacher, he was withdrawn from school and taught by his mother. He later invented the electric light bulb and the phonograph.

Albert Einstein: Teachers considered him to be mentally slow, unsociable and a 'dreamer'. Failed first college entrance examinations, and in the two years after graduation he obtained (and lost!) three teaching positions.

Ultimately he developed the theory of relativity.

Paul Erlich (1854-1915): Completely inept at examinations, he was excused composition writing in college and his thesis was written by a scribe.

He became a famous German bacteriologist, and won a Nobel prize.

Susan Hampshire: Leading stage and screen actress who has appeared on television programmes about dyslexia.

William James: In his book *The Principles of Psychology* he wrote 'I am myself a very poor visualiser and find that I can seldom call to mind a single alphabet letter purely in retinal terms. I must trace the letter by running my mental eye over its contour in order that the image of it shall leave any distinctness at all.'

He was a famous educational psychologist and if the principles that he expressed in his 'talks to teachers on psychology' were followed, many dyslexic students would have little difficulty in capitalising on their abilities, or in learning.

George Patton: Could not read by the age of twelve, and remained deficient in reading all his life. He had, however, an excellent memory and became a famous World War II general.

Nelson Rockefeller: Became vice president of the U.S.A.

Auguste Rodin: Became a pupil of the Jesuit school at which he was educated. An earlier tutor wrote to his father 'He is ineducable. The sooner you put him to work the better.'

He sculpted the classic statue 'The Thinker'.

George Washington: At the age of fourteen, his grammar and spelling was atrocious, but he had a flair for mathematics.

He became a 'Gentleman Farmer' and President of a new nation, the U.S.A.

Woodrow Wilson: Unable to read the alphabet at the age of nine. He was eleven when he learned to read.

He also became a president of the U.S.A.

*   *   *

These are just a few of the people who 'made it' and they have demonstrated that it is possible despite all the odds against them – they must obviously have had great determination.

So how many people might there be, who with a little patient encouragement, might well make worthwhile contributions to the scientific, economic or artistic fields – and to society as a whole?

Books

Spelling Made Easy
V. Brand
Egon Publications, Baldock, 1984
(A series of titles for different age groups)

Development of Dyslexia
Macdonald Critchley
Heinemann, London, 1964

The British Ability Scales
C.D. Elliott and D.J. Murray
NFER-Nelson, Windsor, 1983

Overcoming Dyslexia
B. Hornsby
Macdonald, London, 1984

Help for Dyslexic Children
T.R. Miles and E. Miles
Methuen, London, 1983

Understanding Dyslexia
T.R. Miles and E. Miles
Better Books, Bath, 1986

Checkmate
A Pocket-Sized Guide to Everyday Spellings for Dyslexics
Alan O'Brien
Jessica Kingsley Publishers, London, 1992

Children with Special Needs
Assesment Law and Practice
Caught in the Act
Harry Chasty and John Friel
Jessica Kingsley Publishers, London, 1991

Signposts to Spelling
J. Pollock
Helen Arkell Dyslexia Centre, London, 1978

The School Daze of the Learning Disability Child
W. Silva
Alpern Communications,
220 Gulph Hills Road,
Radnor, PA 19087, U S A

Help for Dyslexic Adults
E.G. Stirling
Better Books, Bath, 1985
(Better Books catalogue contains many useful titles and learning aides and software for Spectrum and BBC 'B')

Journals

Learning Disability Journal (published quarterly)
Department of Special Education
435 Herbert C. Miller Building
University of Kansas Medical Center
Kansas City, Kan 66103

Journal of Learning Disabilities
Professional Press
5 N Wabash Avenue
Chicago, Ill 60602

(Ask at your local reference library for other books)

Useful Addresses
United Kingdom

Advisory Centre for Education
18 Victoria Park Square
London E2 9PB
Tel: (081) 980 4596

British Dyslexia Association
98 London Road
Reading
Berkshire RG1 5AU
Tel: (0734) 668271/2
(A mine of further help and information. Local associations throughout the country – list of addresses available from B.D.A. The Association holds meetings several times a year.)

Dyslexia Institute
133 Gresham Road
Staines
Middlesex TW18 2AJ
Tel: (0784) 63851

Helen Arkell Dyslexia Centre
17 Wandsworth Common West Side
London SW18 2ED
Tel: (081) 871 2846

Learning Development Aids
Duke Street
Wisbech
Cambridgeshire PE13 2AE
Tel. (0945) 63441
(also do lots of books, educational packs, games, software, etc.)

Parents Advice Line
(run by the journal *Special Children*)
Box 161
Rode
Bath
Tel: (0898) 333001

Voluntary Organisations Communication and Language
336 Brixton Road
London SW9
Tel: (071) 274 4029

Many universities now have a department covering
Learning Disabilities. They have access to a great deal of
information and I have found them to be most helpful.

About the author

Michael V. Ryden – born 4th April 1960

Diagnosed as dyslexic by McDonald Critchley (London) in 1969, and then examined by an educational psychologist who reported an IQ rating of well above average. A further test in 1973 confirmed this.

The only help that the local education authority was able to offer at that time was a suggestion that he be sent to a school for the educationally subnormal, as they had no special help available and in fact questioned whether such a thing as dyslexia existed.

After a lot of effort and help he obtained three CSEs, seven GSEs and two GCE 'A' Level grades in examinations, GSE grade four being the highest in English and maths and physics being taken at 'A' Level.

He took a course in Business Studies and learned a great deal although he failed the final examinations because of poor English grades.

He could not gain entrance to university in the United Kingdom because of his English grades, but was fortunate enough to go to a university in the United States of America where he obtained a BSc in Photography and Graphics.

He is now starting a career in photography.